UNDERSTANDING GLUCOSE REVOLUTION

Discover the Transformative Effect of Blood Sugar Harmony, Healthy Glucose Level, Preventing Diseases, Wellness and Longevity

BRUCE BOWSER

All rights reserved. No part of this publication may be reproduced, distributed, or transmitted in any form or by any means, including photocopying, recording, or other electronic or mechanical methods, without the prior written permission of the publisher, except in the case of brief quotations embodied in critical reviews and certain other noncommercial uses permitted by copyright law.

Copyright © Bruce Bowser, 2024

INTRODUCTION: 5
UNDERSTANDING GLUCOSE Significance and Functions   5

CHAPTER 1   23
THE BOTANICAL ALCHEMY: UNVEILING THE SECRETS OF PLANT-MADE GLUCOSE   23
    CAN THE HUMAN BODY MAKE GLUCOSE?   27

CHAPTER 2   31
THE PATH TO CIRCULATION: Tracing the journey of Glucose into the Bloodstream.   31

CHAPTER 3   37
MODERN DIETS: 37
The Surge in Glucose Consumption Over-Time   37
    The Obesity Epidemic   41
    Impact on Health: Obesity and Metabolic Disorders - Unraveling the Consequences of Excessive Glucose Consumption   60

CHAPTER 4   81
UNRAVELING THE GLUCOSE SURGE: 81
Exploring the Phenomenon of Spikes   81
    What Is High Blood Sugar?   89
    What Are the Symptoms of a Blood Sugar Spike?   90
        Symptoms of Diabetic Ketoacidosis   94
    What Are the Causes of Blood Sugar Spikes?   95

How to Manage Blood Sugar 97
How to Prevent Blood Sugar Spikes 105
Long-term side effects 107

CHAPTER 5 — 115
THE TRIAD OF EFFECTS — 115
Deconstructing the Three Consequences of Glucose Spikes — 115

Insulin Resistance: A Crescendo of Metabolic Disruption 116

The Interplay of Consequences: A Symphony of Metabolic Challenges 119

CHAPTER 6 — 121
MASTERING THE ART OF BLOOD SUGAR BALANCE — 121
Strategies to Level Your Glucose Curve — 121

CHAPTER 7 — 130
DIABETES NUTRITIONAL GUIDE — 130
What is the glycemic index (GI)? — 130

What factors affect a food's glycemic index rating? 134

What are the benefits of using the glycemic index? 140

What are the risks of eating on the glycemic index? 141

The glycemic index of common fruits and vegetables 143

Takeaway 152

INTRODUCTION:

UNDERSTANDING GLUCOSE
Significance and Functions

Glucose, a simple sugar, serves as a fundamental building block of life and plays a pivotal role in various physiological processes within the human body.

The Greek word meaning "sweet" is where the word "glucose" originates. Your body uses this type of sugar, which it obtains from the food you eat, as fuel. When it enters your circulation and travels to your cells, it is known as blood glucose or blood sugar.

A hormone called insulin moves glucose from the circulation into cells where it is stored and used as fuel.

The primary source of glucose is carbohydrate-rich foods like bread, potatoes, and fruit. When you eat, food travels from your oesophagus to your stomach. There, it is broken down into little pieces by acids and enzymes. During this procedure, glucose is released.

It gets absorbed once it reaches your intestines. After that, it is absorbed into your bloodstream. Once in the circulation, insulin facilitates the delivery of glucose to your cells.

The Essential Role of Glucose
Why does glucose play such a significant role in the vast web of human biology? Its

ability to serve as the main energy source for our cells holds the key to the answer. Our body's energy system, which includes the mitochondria, the cell's power plant, and the intricate web of neurons firing in our brain, prefers to run on glucose.

Apart from being an energy source, glucose serves as an essential component in the synthesis of complex molecules. It contributes to the synthesis of lipids, proteins, and nucleic acids, which means it is crucial for the upkeep and development of our cells.

The Dance of Hormones: Regulating Glucose Levels

Comprehending glucose involves not only identifying its existence but also deciphering the complex hormonal dance that regulates its concentration. Insulin and glucagon, the dynamic duo of the endocrine system, precisely balance each other out to keep glucose levels within a narrow, optimal range. The chaos that would result from too big or too small fluctuations in glucose concentrations is avoided by this careful balancing.

ENERGY AND STORAGE

Your body is designed to keep the level of glucose in your blood constant. Your pancreas's beta cells check your blood sugar level every few seconds. After eating, as blood glucose levels rise, beta cells release insulin into the bloodstream. Insulin acts as a key, allowing glucose to enter by opening the cells of the liver, muscle, and fat.

The majority of cells in your body use lipids, carbohydrates, and amino acids (which are the building blocks of proteins) as fuel. It is your brain's main source of food, nevertheless. Information processing is necessary for nerve cells and chemical messengers. Without it, your brain could not operate as it should.

Your body stores the leftover glucose in tiny bundles called glycogen in your muscles and liver after using all of the energy it needs. About a day's worth of energy may be stored in your body.

After several hours without food, your blood sugar level returns to normal. The pancreas stops generating insulin. The pancreatic alpha cells start to produce glucagon, a different hormone. It gives the liver instructions to break down glycogen stores and converts it back to glucose.

This gets into your circulation and fills you full until the next time you have food. Additionally, your liver can make glucose on its own from lipids, amino acids, and waste products.

Gluconeogenesis

The liver and kidneys participate in gluconeogenesis, a process that creates glucose from non-carbohydrate precursors, during periods of fasting or low glucose availability. This maintains the general metabolic balance by guaranteeing a constant supply of glucose to essential organs.

Glucose and Brain Function

Glucose is very important to the brain as an energy source. Since glucose is the main fuel for brain activity, changes in its availability may have an effect on cognitive performance. The blood-brain barrier controls the amount of glucose that enters the brain, highlighting the vital role that glucose plays in preserving cognitive function.

Sugar's Role in Health and Illness

It's not all sunshine and honey in the story of glucose. Its control can become unbalanced, with disastrous results possible, most notably diabetes.

After eating, your blood sugar usually increases. After insulin delivers glucose to your cells a few hours later, it falls. Between meals, your blood sugar should be less than 100 mg/dl, or milligrams per deciliter. We call this your fasting blood sugar level.

Diabetes Mellitus

Health problems can arise from imbalances in glucose metabolism, diabetes mellitus being one well-known example. Hyperglycemia is the outcome of the body's inability to control blood glucose levels in people with diabetes. In order to control and prevent diabetes, it is essential to comprehend the complex interactions between insulin, glucagon, and glucose metabolism.

re two types of diabetes

A person with type 1 diabetes has insufficient insulin in their body. The cells of the pancreas, which produces insulin, are attacked and destroyed by the immune system.

The cells in type 2 diabetes don't react to insulin as they ought to. In order to transfer glucose into the cells, the pancreas must produce an increasing amount of insulin. The pancreas eventually suffers damage and is unable to produce enough insulin to fulfill the body's requirements.

An inadequate amount of insulin prevents glucose from entering cells. The blood sugar level doesn't go down. When blood glucose levels are higher than 200 mg/dl two hours after a meal or 125 mg/dl when fasting, it is called hyperglycemia.

Over time, high blood glucose levels can damage the arteries that carry oxygen-rich blood to your organs. Elevated blood sugar levels can increase your chance of:

- Cardiovascular illness, heart attack, and stroke
- Kidney failure
- Damage to the nerves
- Retinopathy is a kind of eye illness.

Regular blood sugar testing is necessary for diabetics. To prevent these problems and maintain blood glucose levels in a healthy range, three main strategies can be used: exercise, diet, and medication.

HYPOGLYCEMIA (Low blood sugar)

Often known as low blood sugar, hypoglycemia is a medical disease marked by unusually low blood glucose levels. Although the body needs glucose as an energy source, an imbalance in the molecule's levels can cause a range of symptoms, from minor discomfort to serious consequences. The causes, symptoms, and treatment options for hypoglycemia are covered in this chapter.

Causes of Hypoglycemia

- Excessive Insulin

An abundance of insulin in the blood is one of the main reasons for hypoglycemia. When people with diabetes use insulin or certain oral drugs to control their blood sugar levels, this frequently happens. Insulin helps cells absorb glucose, and too much of it can cause blood sugar levels to decrease sharply.

- Missed or delayed meals

Hypoglycemia can result from irregular eating schedules or meal skipping. Low blood sugar can occur from the body not getting enough glucose on a regular basis, particularly in those with diabetes or those using blood sugar-lowering drugs.

- Alcohol Consumption

Drinking too much alcohol might affect the body's capacity to control blood sugar levels. Alcohol consumption can affect the liver's ability to release glucose into the circulation, which can result in hypoglycemia, particularly in diabetics.

- Certain medications

Hypoglycemia is a possible adverse effect of several drugs, such as those used to treat specific illnesses or disorders. People who take drugs need to talk to their healthcare professionals and be aware of any possible interactions.

Symptoms of Hypoglycemia

- Shakiness and Tremors

Sheer trembling is one of the first symptoms of hypoglycemia. This happens when the body releases stress chemicals like adrenaline in reaction to low blood sugar.

- Perspiration and Sickness

Among the most typical signs of hypoglycemia are excessive perspiration and clammy skin. During a hypoglycemic episode, the body attempts to regulate its temperature, which results in excessive sweating.

- Confusion and Irritability

Low blood sugar levels can impair cognitive function, resulting in agitation, disorientation, and trouble focusing. Both interpersonal connections and day-to-day activities may be impacted by these symptoms.

- Dizziness and Weakness

During hypoglycemia, people frequently report feeling weak or dizzy. This may make it difficult to do daily duties and increase the chance of falling.

- Loss of Consciousness

Untreated hypoglycemia can cause coma, convulsions, and loss of consciousness in extreme circumstances. Promptly treating hypoglycemia is essential to avoiding these potentially fatal consequences.

Management of Hypoglycemia

- Immediate Glucose Intake

Eating a fast-absorbing glucose source is the best strategy for treating hypoglycemia. This can include gel, glucose pills, or meals like fruit juice or candies that contain simple sugar.

- Regular Monitoring

People who have diabetes or who are susceptible to hypoglycemia should check their blood sugar levels often. This makes it easier to see trends and modify lifestyle choices or prescriptions as necessary.

- Balanced Diet and Meal Timing

Eating regular, well-timed meals and sticking to a balanced diet will help avoid hypoglycemia spells. Meals high in proteins, healthy fats, and complex carbs release glucose into the circulation gradually.

- Medication Adjustments

Hypoglycemia in diabetics can be avoided by modifying insulin or medicine dosages in cooperation with medical professionals. Finding the ideal balance is essential for successful blood sugar management.

Careful treatment of hypoglycemia is necessary to avoid problems and enhance general health. Maintaining ideal blood sugar levels requires identifying the reasons, identifying the symptoms, and putting preventative and treatment plans into practice. People who are at risk of hypoglycemia, especially those who have diabetes, should collaborate closely with their medical team to create a customized strategy that takes into account their unique requirements and lifestyle choices.

Glucose has far more importance and uses than just being a basic sugar. Glucose is essential to the complex web of life because it powers cellular functions, maintains homeostasis, and enhances cognitive function. Understanding glucose and its metabolism thoroughly is crucial for deciphering the enigmas of human physiology and creating strategies for promoting health and preventing diseases.

CHAPTER 1

THE BOTANICAL ALCHEMY:
UNVEILING THE SECRETS OF PLANT-MADE GLUCOSE

The mechanism by which plants make food is called photosynthesis. Their leaves are the first to collect light energy, carbon dioxide from the atmosphere, and water from the soil. Water oxidizes, carbon dioxide is lowered, and electrons are acquired within plant cells. In the process, carbon dioxide is changed into glucose and water into oxygen. While the energy is stored in glucose molecules, the oxygen is released into the environment.

For plants to develop, flourish, and make other substances like cellulose and starch, they require this energy. While cellulose is utilized by these plants to produce cell walls, starch is stored in plant parts and seeds for use as a food source. Starches may be found in foods like rice and wheat.

To put it simply, a complicated series of chemical reactions known as photosynthesis uses water, carbon dioxide, and oxygen from sunlight to create glucose, a simple sugar.

But not every type of photosynthesis is the same. The majority of plants use carbon three (C3) to create 3-phosphoglyceric acid, a three-carbon compound that eventually produces glucose. A plant's kind of photosynthesis is dictated by the resources found in its surroundings. For instance, C4 photosynthesis produces more carbon and enables plants to flourish in environments with limited light and water.

Chlorophyll is a pigment or substance that is found in most plants on Earth and is used by them for photosynthesis. Solar energy is captured by this chlorophyll and converted to chemical energy. The leaves seem green because it reflects green light from the sun and absorbs blue and red light. As they cease producing chlorophyll, plants' leaves change color, as we can observe in the fall.

Chloroplasts are small organelles that are present in plant cells and can contain chlorophyll. Broccoli and green zucchini are two examples of plant-based foods that are high in this vitamin. A food is greener the more chlorophyll it contains. All plants contain either or both of the two types of chlorophyll: chlorophyll a and chlorophyll b. Both varieties of chlorophyll are fat-soluble molecules that also have antioxidant characteristics.

CAN THE HUMAN BODY MAKE GLUCOSE?

Think of your body as a skilled chef in a busy kitchen, always in the mood to create the ideal energy recipe. Your body is the chef in this gourmet adventure, and it has an amazing talent: it can make glucose, the body's favorite fuel, out of unexpected sources.

Your body doesn't give up when your stomach is rumbling and there are no groceries in the pantry. Rather, it uses a clever process called gluconeogenesis, which is the art of creating glucose in the kitchen.

Think of your liver as the head chef and your body as the kitchen. Let's now examine the components that are available:

Amino Acids - The Proteins:

Proteins are like building bricks in the refrigerator (your body's cells), just waiting to be used. The chef extracts the amino acids from these proteins and converts them to glucose when energy is required. It's similar to creating a gourmet dish out of leftovers.

Lactate - The Workout Byproduct:

Consider lactate to be the perspiration-producing result of your muscles working hard during a strenuous exercise session. Your body transfers it to the liver, where it gets a culinary makeover and becomes part of the glucose recipe, instead of wasting it. This is the best kind of recycling.

Glycerol - The Fat Breakdown Component:

Now see your body's stored fats as the olive oil on the shelf. One of these lipids, glycerol, moves forward when the body needs glucose. It's similar to making a delicious sauce using pantry oil.

The chef creates a symphony of biochemical events when these materials come together in the liver, which functions as a type of molecular kitchen. It's an evolved survival strategy, a sensible reaction to the body's need for energy.

The hormones perform the tasks of kitchen helpers: glucagon, which encourages the chef to increase glucose production when necessary, and insulin, which acts as a regulator to keep dishes from being too sweet.

Can the human body produce glucose then? Indeed. It's just a regular cooking routine, nothing fancy or exotic. You may be confident that your body's internal chef is working hard to keep the energy pot boiling by creating the perfect quantity of glucose when your body's pantry runs short.

CHAPTER 2

THE PATH TO CIRCULATION:
Tracing the journey of Glucose into the Bloodstream.

Understanding the complex interaction between the food we consume and the energy our bodies make from it requires an understanding of how glucose enters the circulation. This chapter offers a fascinating tour of the metabolic pathways that control the fate of glucose, emphasizing the crucial intervals between absorption and ingestion.

Think of your body as a busy kitchen, where the delectable spread on your plate signals the start of a wonderful gastronomic adventure. Here, in this appetizer, we dissect the complex mechanisms of digestion and absorption, much like a chef preparing and serving a delicious dish.

The Feast on Your Plate: Diverse Carbohydrates

During a meal, different types of carbohydrates become prominent. Every element, be it the simplicity of sugars, the coziness of starches, or the sweetness of fruits, adds to the overall taste experience. We have no idea that hidden away in this delicious treat is glucose, the body's energy currency—a simple but vital substance.

Gastronomic Alchemy: Digestion in the Stomach

The voyage of taste commences in the stomach, where the digestive system starts its alchemical conversion. Enzymes in this case convert complicated carbs into simpler sugars, such as glucose, the main player in this story. It is similar to a chef carefully chopping components to bring out the tastes of a meal.

Small Intestine: Absorption

The trip then takes us to the first step of absorption, the small intestine. Imagine the walls of the small intestine covered in microscopic projections that resemble fingers, called villi. Like gourmet chefs, these villi improve the absorption of nutrients, including glucose. By these actions, glucose enters the circulation and moves from the digestive to the circulatory phases.

Portal Vein: The Culinary Highway to the Liver

Now that glucose has entered the circulation, it travels the portal vein, a culinary route. This specific pathway takes one straight to the liver, the culinary maestro of metabolism in our bodies. Here, glucose is given many options: it can be released straight into the bloodstream to meet urgent energy demands, stored as glycogen for later use, or transformed into lipids.

Circulation of Blood: A Sophisticated Symphony

Glucose enters the bloodstream and travels through it like a musical instrument. Glucose is transported throughout the body in a rhythmic manner by the heartbeat. It reaches a variety of "tables," such as neurons and muscle cells, supplying the energy needs of all tissues.

Regulatory Chefs: Insulin and Glucagon

Hormones such as glucagon and insulin are the regulatory cooks in this gastronomic drama. The pancreas secretes insulin, which directs cells' absorption of glucose and therefore lowers blood sugar levels. On the other hand, when the body needs an extra energy boost, glucagon causes the liver to release glucose that has been stored. The hormonal dance keeps the culinary orchestra in a precise balance.

We see the wonders of the body's culinary dance as we follow the path of glucose into the circulation. From the first delicious meal to the absorption in the small intestine to the circulatory circulation, this gourmet journey reflects the smooth manner in which the body coordinates the transit and consumption of glucose, the necessary component for powering life's culinary processes.

CHAPTER 3

MODERN DIETS:

The Surge in Glucose Consumption Over-Time

The last century has seen a significant change in how humans ingest and metabolize glucose within the constantly changing realm of dietary practices. The growth in sedentary lifestyles, the expansion of processed foods, and modifications to farming techniques have all contributed to a notable rise in the intake of glucose. This chapter explores the causes of this increase and how it affects people's health.

The Rise of Processed Foods: A Culinary Revolution with Health Implications

A revolutionary change in the production, distribution, and consumption of food has characterized the evolution of dietary patterns throughout the 20th and 21st centuries. Leading this gastronomic revolution is the extraordinary surge in processed food consumption, which has altered our dietary habits and, therefore, significantly impacted the way our bodies metabolize glucose.

The Convenience Paradigm:

The growing popularity of processed meals is directly related to our fast-paced, modern society's need for convenience. Packaged snacks, prepared meals, and sugary drinks have proliferated, providing convenient options for people managing hectic schedules. Convenience generally comes at the expense of nutritional content, since processed meals often include high levels of refined sugars and carbs.

Hidden Sugars and Sweeteners:

It's well known that processed foods include unrecognized sugars and sweeteners. These added sugars, which contribute to an overabundance of readily digested carbs, go by a variety of names on ingredient lists, such as sucrose, high fructose corn syrup, and other syrups. These hidden sugars raise the amount of glucose in our meals and make it harder to manage blood sugar. They may be found in anything from salad dressings to morning cereals.

Impact on Blood Sugar Levels:

The rapid absorption of carbs in processed meals may cause blood glucose levels to rise. Unlike the gradual release of sugars from natural foods, the concentrated sugars in processed meals flood the circulation and trigger an insulin response. Over time, this loop may make insulin resistance worse, which is a significant risk factor for type 2 diabetes.

Refined Carbohydrates and Glycemic Index:

Many processed meals include refined carbs, which have a high glycemic index.

Because these carbohydrates break down quickly into glucose, blood sugar levels increase quickly and are often overestimated. A regular diet high in carbs may lead to insulin resistance and metabolic problems.

The Obesity Epidemic

Processed food consumption is increasing worldwide in tandem with rising obesity rates. These meals, which are frequently high in energy and low in nutrients, add to an excessive consumption of calories. When excess energy is not used up via exercise, it is stored as fat, which raises the risk of issues associated with obesity, such as insulin resistance and type 2 diabetes.

Addressing the Challenge:

Although processed foods are convenient and palatable, a collective change in dietary choices is necessary to overcome the problems they provide to glucose metabolism. People can be more equipped to make educated decisions, read food labels, and navigate the current food environment in a healthier way if they get education on these topics.

The emergence of processed foods has brought about a shift in dietary practices that has a significant effect on how we use glucose. Understanding the effects of this change and advocating for a return to whole, unprocessed foods are crucial to reducing the health concerns brought on by the spike in glucose intake and to encouraging a sustainable, balanced diet.

Changing Agricultural Practices: Harvesting Glucose in the Modern Fields

The structure of contemporary agriculture has changed dramatically, which has a variety of effects on how our foods are made and, in turn, how our bodies metabolize carbohydrates. Alterations in agricultural practices, ranging from crop selection to farming methods, have significantly influenced the nutritional composition of the meals we eat.

Monoculture and Depletion of Nutrients:

A prominent change in farming methods is the increasing occurrence of mono-cropping, in which large areas of land are planted with only one type of crop. Although this technique works well for large-scale production, the soil frequently loses nutrients as a result of it. Crops may thus have lower concentrations of important minerals, such as magnesium and chromium, which are involved in the metabolism of glucose.

Hybridization and Increased Sugar Content:

Hybrid cultivars have been developed as a result of the drive for higher crop production and pest resistance. These types could be more resilient, although occasionally they have more sugar content. For instance, the natural sugar content of some fruits and vegetables may be higher than others, which causes the body to absorb more glucose when ingested.

Genetic Modification and Modified Ratios of Nutrients:

The nutritional content of crops has been further modified by the introduction of genetic manipulation in agriculture. Even though the goal of these adjustments is frequently to improve traits like insect resistance, they may unintentionally alter nutritional ratios. A disturbance in the balance of vital nutrients that are involved in the control of glucose levels might affect the overall effect of meals on blood sugar levels.

Pesticides and Their Impact on Metabolism:

Concerns have been raised concerning the possible effects of pesticides on human health despite their widespread usage in contemporary agriculture to protect crops from diseases and pests.

According to certain research, there may be a link between exposure to pesticides and abnormalities in metabolic functions, which might affect how the body uses glucose. Research on the complex interactions between agricultural chemicals and human metabolism is still underway.

Soil Microbiome and Nutrients Absorption:

Crop nutrition is closely related to the condition of the soil microbiome, a complex population of microorganisms in the soil. Alterations in farming methods, such as applying artificial fertilizers and pesticides, may have an effect on the variety and well-being of the soil microbiota. Consequently, this might impact the nutrients' bioavailability that are essential for the metabolism of glucose.

Sustainable Agriculture and Nutrient-Rich Foods:

In spite of these obstacles, people are becoming more conscious of the significance of sustainable farming methods. Regenerative agriculture is one practice that emphasizes nutrient-rich crops, biodiversity, and healthy soil. Selecting foods produced sustainably might result in a better nutritional profile and possibly improve glucose metabolism.

The way that agriculture is evolving affects the nutrients that are in the food we eat and, in turn, how our systems handle glucose. In order to create a future in which agricultural decisions enhance general health and well-being, it might be crucial to recognize the complexity of these interactions and to promote sustainable farming methods.

Sedentary Lifestyles and Insulin Resistance: The Modern Challenge to Glucose Metabolism

We live in a unique age when sedentary tendencies have become the norm due to the influence of technology and ease. Long-term inactivity has consequences that go beyond poor physical health; they include a significant influence on the metabolism of glucose and the emergence of insulin resistance, which is a crucial step on the path to metabolic diseases.

The Dilemma of the Desk-Bound:

The sedentary nature of modern companies, which sometimes restrict people to desks and computers, contrasts sharply with the physically active lifestyles of bygone eras. Sedentary activities such as spending a lot of time in front of computers or sitting in workplaces raise the risk of insulin resistance.

Physical Inactivity and Glucose Uptake:

Maintaining insulin sensitivity—the body's capacity to use insulin and control blood glucose levels—requires regular physical exercise.

The muscles' capacity to absorb glucose decreases with less physical activity, which is the situation with sedentary lives. Over time, this decrease in glucose absorption may contribute to insulin resistance by raising blood sugar levels.

Adipose Tissue and Inflammation:

Visceral fat, especially in the belly, can accumulate as a result of sedentary lifestyles. This kind of fat promotes a long-term state of low-grade inflammation because it is metabolically active and produces inflammatory chemicals. Insulin resistance is thus encouraged by inflammation's interference with insulin signaling pathways.

Impact on Mitochondrial Function:

Increased mitochondrial function—the engine of our cells that produces energy—is linked to regular physical activity. Conversely, sedentary activity may reduce the effectiveness of the mitochondria. Insulin resistance is made worse by disruptions in energy metabolism, which are caused by diminished mitochondrial activity.

The Role of Screen Time:

The popularity of screen-based work and leisure has greatly increased the incidence of sedentary activities. Long hours spent on computers and cellphones, or binge-watching television shows, are associated with longer screen times and lower levels of physical activity. Increased insulin resistance and a greater risk of type 2 diabetes are associated with this lifestyle factor.

Breaking the Sedentary Cycle:

Sedentary lifestyles provide a number of difficulties that require a multimodal strategy to address. Insulin sensitivity can be enhanced by incorporating regular physical activity into everyday activities, such as walking, cycling, or participating in organized exercise. Furthermore, implementing brief rest intervals between extended periods of sitting has been demonstrated to improve glucose metabolism.

Public Health Initiatives:

Since sedentary behaviors have negative effects on public health, programs that encourage physical exercise have gained popularity. Initiatives for community fitness, workplace wellness, and education all stress the value of an active lifestyle in reducing insulin resistance and associated metabolic illnesses.

Sedentary lifestyles are a contemporary problem that affect glucose metabolism and lead to the development of insulin resistance. Recognizing the effects of extended periods of inactivity and implementing tactics to incorporate physical exercise back into everyday life are essential measures to protect metabolic health and stop the development of diseases like type 2 diabetes.

Hidden Sugars in Foods: Unveiling the Sweet Culprits of Modern Diets

Sweets entice us across the board in our diets, not just in the dessert section. Hiding in many common meals are hidden sugars, a more subtle cause than the apparent candy and sugary drinks. To fully comprehend these hidden sweeteners' effects on glucose metabolism and general health, it is imperative to uncover their widespread use.

- Disguised Delight:

Concealed behind pseudonyms such as sucrose, agave nectar, or high-fructose corn syrup, hidden sugars are skilled at disguising themselves as sweet ingredients in meals so they may not be noticed as such. Savory sauces and even supposedly healthful granola bars can have unexpectedly high sugar contents, which adds to the bloodstream's continuous flow of glucose.

The Sneaky Nature of Added Sugars:

Sugars are often added to processed and packaged meals in order to improve flavor, increase shelf life, or make the product more pleasant. It can be difficult for consumers to recognize and regulate their sugar intake since products like flavored yogurts, breakfast cereals, and even seemingly harmless condiments may have added sugars.

Impacts on Blood Sugar Levels:

Stable blood sugar regulation is significantly hampered by hidden sugars' clandestine nature. Added sugars have the potential to cause abrupt increases and subsequent drops in blood sugar, in contrast to natural sugars present in whole fruits and unprocessed diets. Over time, this irregular pattern may exacerbate insulin resistance by stressing the body's insulin response.

The Unhealthy Alliance: Processed Foods and Hidden Sugars:

A recurring motif in contemporary diets is the union of processed foods with hidden sugars. Convenience meals that appear benign, sweetened drinks, and processed snacks can all have surprisingly high added sugar content. The fact that sugar is addicting adds to the difficulty by starting a vicious cycle of seeking and consumption that feeds the underlying sugar problem.

The Impact on Overall Health:

Overindulgence in hidden sugars has negative health effects that extend beyond glucose metabolism. Sugar additions give empty calories, which raise the risk of metabolic diseases, weight gain, and obesity. A diet heavy in unrecognized sugars is also linked to cardiovascular problems, inflammation, and a higher chance of type 2 diabetes.

Unmasking Hidden Sugars: Reading Labels and Making Informed Choices:

One must have an excellent eye for reading food labels in order to empower people to make educated decisions. It's essential to know the many labels for hidden sugars and to spot them in ingredient lists. People may better control their blood sugar levels by consuming less packaged goods and choosing whole, unprocessed meals. This will help them take charge of their sugar intake.

Public Awareness and Health Advocacy:

A critical first step in tackling the problem at a societal level is raising public awareness of the prevalence of hidden sugars. Together, health advocacy efforts, nutritional education programs, and legislation governing food labeling control food safety and encourage the use of healthier foods.

Hidden sugars weave themselves into the fabric of modern diets, posing a significant challenge to glucose metabolism and overall health. Unmasking these sweet culprits requires a vigilant approach to food choices, a commitment to reading labels, and a broader societal effort to foster awareness and promote healthier eating habits.

Impact on Health: Obesity and Metabolic Disorders - Unraveling the Consequences of Excessive Glucose Consumption

Increased intake of glucose, especially from processed foods and hidden sugars, is a major factor in the health story that is still being written. It frequently leads to the complex chapters on obesity and metabolic diseases. A critical viewpoint on the wider effects of contemporary food trends can be gained by comprehending the consequences of high glucose levels.

The cascade of obesity:

Overabundance of blood glucose, particularly when it is not immediately used as fuel, plays a major role in the emergence of obesity. The extra glucose is turned into fat and stored in adipose tissue when the body's cells reach a point where they can no longer store it. In addition to causing weight gain, this adipose buildup prepares the ground for a series of metabolic problems.

Insulin Resistance and Type 2 Diabetes:

Increased blood sugar and obesity are frequently associated with insulin resistance, a disorder in which cells lose their sensitivity to the actions of insulin. In an effort to make up for the body's difficulties controlling blood sugar, the pancreas increases insulin production. The chronic combination of high insulin and poor glucose management raises the risk of type 2 diabetes over time.

Metabolic Syndrome:

The phrase "metabolic syndrome" encapsulates the convergence of insulin resistance, dysregulated glucose metabolism, and obesity. This group of illnesses considerably increases the risk of type 2 diabetes and cardiovascular disease.

It comprises high blood pressure, abnormal cholesterol, and extra belly fat. One real effect of the current nutritional environment is the emergence of metabolic syndrome.

Cardiovascular Implications:

Overindulgence in glucose affects cardiovascular health in addition to metabolic factors. Atherosclerosis, hypertension, and other cardiovascular problems are more likely to occur in people who are obese and have metabolic disorders.

Increased blood sugar levels worsen the integrity of the cardiovascular system by causing oxidative stress and inflammation.

Oxidative Stress and Inflammation:

Chronically consuming large amounts of glucose, particularly from refined and processed foods, causes the body to become inflamed. When combined with oxidative stress, this chronic inflammatory state creates the conditions for a host of health problems. Inflammation is essential to the course of metabolic diseases and is intimately associated with the emergence of insulin resistance.

Liver and Pancreatic Challenges:

Overindulgence in glucose takes a toll on the liver and pancreas, two organs essential to glucose metabolism. Fat infiltration into the liver can result in non-alcoholic fatty liver disease

(NAFLD), and the pancreas can eventually get exhausted from producing insulin continuously. Each situation plays a part in the intricate interaction between metabolic disruptions.

The importance of public health

The increasing prevalence of metabolic diseases and obesity highlight the need for a public health emergency. To address the underlying causes of these health issues, it is imperative to implement policies that support better food environments, nutritional education, and lifestyle interventions. Campaigns to raise public knowledge are essential for enabling people to make decisions regarding their diets and general well-being.

Overconsumption of glucose has a complex effect on health, with metabolic diseases and obesity being major chapters in the story. Modern food trends provide a number of issues that must be addressed with a comprehensive strategy that includes community interventions, individual lifestyle decisions, and larger social initiatives to promote a culture of health and well-being.

The Role of Dietary Choices: Navigating the Path to Optimal Glucose Metabolism

Dietary decisions become the director of the show that takes place within our bodies in the complex dance of glucose metabolism. Not only may the meals we choose satisfy our appetite, but they also have the ability to alter the delicate balance of glucose levels. A road map for promoting ideal metabolic health is provided by realizing the critical significance that food decisions play.

Balancing Carbohydrates:

Glucose mostly comes from carbohydrates, especially from whole, unprocessed sources. Choosing complex carbs means that the bloodstream will release glucose more gradually and steadily—think whole grains, legumes, and veggies. This well-rounded strategy helps to maintain steady energy levels throughout the day by preventing abrupt blood sugar spikes and drops.

Embracing Fiber-Rich Foods:

In terms of dietary decisions, fiber is an unsung hero that is essential to glucose metabolism. Fiber, which is rich in whole grains, legumes, fruits, and vegetables, slows down the absorption of glucose and provides bulk to the diet. This steady release promotes general metabolic health and helps to keep blood sugar levels stable.

Incorporating Healthy Fats:

Nutritional fat is not the evil that the media previously made it out to be. Nuts, seeds, avocados, and olive oil are good sources of healthy fats that help control glucose metabolism and promote fullness. Consuming these fats in the diet helps reduce the sharp spike in blood sugar that is frequently brought on by high-carb meals and offers a source of long-lasting energy.

Prioritizing Lean Proteins:

In addition to being the building elements of the body, proteins are involved in the control of blood sugar. Lean protein foods, such fish, chicken, tofu, and lentils, assist control blood sugar levels by reducing the rate at which carbs are absorbed and digested. To keep metabolism in balance, macronutrient balance is essential.

Mindful Eating Practices:

Eating habits are important, in addition to the makeup of the food. Observing our hunger cues, enjoying every bite, and realizing when we are full are all parts of mindful eating. By encouraging a healthy connection with food, this strategy helps regulate weight and avoid overindulgence, two important aspects of glucose metabolism.

Reducing Sugary and Processed Foods:

Processed meals loaded with unrecognized sugars are a common sight in the modern diet. Glucose levels can be considerably impacted by making deliberate decisions to reduce the consumption of sugary snacks, sweetened beverages, and highly processed meals. A more glucose-friendly diet includes reading product labels, comprehending ingredient lists, and favoring natural foods over packaged ones.

Customizing Diets for Individual Needs:

Given the variety of people and their distinct metabolic reactions, it's critical to customize diets to meet the demands of each individual. The body metabolizes glucose differently depending on age, exercise level, and underlying medical disorders, among other factors. Seeking advice from certified dietitians or medical specialists can offer tailored recommendations for creating the ideal diet.

Culinary Exploration and Variety:

Consuming a wide range of nutrient-dense meals not only guarantees a spectrum of vital nutrients but also enhances the taste experience. Diverse culinary explorations, novel recipe development, and the inclusion of a rainbow of fruits and vegetables in meals may promote a vibrant and fulfilling approach to nutrition.

The Long-Term Commitment to Health:

Making healthy food choices is a long-term commitment to wellbeing rather than a quick cure. A lifestyle that promotes optimal glucose metabolism and general health can be achieved by forming enduring habits, progressively introducing healthful foods into daily routines, and adhering to a balanced nutritional plan.

Dietary decisions have the effect of a conductor directing a symphony of metabolic events in relation to glucose metabolism. Giving people the ability to make thoughtful, customized, and educated food decisions creates the conditions for a harmonious interaction of nutrients and, in the end, aids the body's path to ideal glucose metabolism and general health.

Future Perspectives: Redefining Diets for Health - Navigating Towards a Glucose-Friendly Future

We are at a turning point in the evolution of nutrition, and how food trends develop in the future might fundamentally alter how we think about health and well-being. Future diet definitions will involve a comprehensive investigation of sustainable options, advancements in technology, and a more profound comprehension of the complex relationships between nutrition and metabolic health.

Embracing Sustainable Nutrition:

Sustainability is inextricably tied to diets in the future, for the sake of both human and environmental health. Plant-based diets that emphasize a range of fruits, vegetables, legumes, and whole grains not only enhance metabolic health but also help maintain the sustainability of the ecosystem. The trend toward plant-centric diets is in line with the rising understanding of how dietary decisions affect one's own health as well as the health of the world at large.

Personalized Nutrition and Nutrigenomics:

Nutrigenomics research is making it possible to create individualized diet programs based on each person's unique genetic makeup. Food recommendations that maximize metabolic health may be made with accuracy when one understands the precise interactions between an individual's distinct genetic makeup and dietary choices. Personalized approaches are the key to better glucose control and general health initiatives.

Innovation in Nutrition and Technology:

Creative solutions are being made possible by the use of technology into the field of nutrition. Technology is emerging as a useful ally in the pursuit of ideal glucose metabolism, from wearable gadgets that track real-time metabolic data to smart kitchen equipment that assist in meal preparation. People are becoming more capable of making educated food decisions because of digital platforms, apps, and continuous glucose monitors that provide customized nutrition information.

The Rise of Functional Foods:

Functional meals are becoming more and more popular since they are made to offer particular health advantages in addition to vital nutrients. Foods are becoming more and more filled with prebiotics, probiotics, and bioactive substances to improve metabolic function, control inflammation, and promote gut health. Diets in the future could place more emphasis on foods that actively support metabolic health in addition to providing nourishment.

Integrating Traditional Wisdom:

There's a newfound regard for time-tested traditional food habits in the pursuit of dietary evolution. Culturally inspired diets frequently place an emphasis on seasonal fluctuations and whole, minimally processed foods. These old diets may become more popular in the future as people realize how wise they are in terms of supporting metabolic and nutritional health.

Educating and Empowering:
Future dietary paradigms will emphasize nutritional empowerment and knowledge

more than ever. It will be essential to comprehend the principles of nutrition, read food labels, and have a greater understanding of how dietary decisions affect metabolic health. Accessible materials and educational programs will be essential in helping people develop more knowledgeable and responsible eating habits.

Promoting Wholesome Health:

Diets in the future will involve a comprehensive approach to health rather than just a list of items to eat. A whole approach to metabolic health must include stress management, regular physical exercise, enough sleep, and mindful eating habits. The diets of the future will emphasize the interrelated aspects of mental, emotional, and physical well-being in addition to providing nourishment for the body.

Collaborative Efforts for Change:

Redefining diets for health is a move that calls for cooperation on many levels. The future of diets is a collaborative effort including everyone from people making educated decisions to legislators putting policies for better food environments into action.

A paradigm change in dietary perspectives will be facilitated by the creation of supporting legislation, the promotion of sustainable farming methods, and the advocacy for nutritional education.

Diets may undergo a paradigm change in the future, moving away from traditional beliefs and toward a more enlightened and comprehensive view of health. We have the opportunity to transform our relationship with food and create a future where diets not only promote normal glucose metabolism but also feed the body by embracing sustainability, utilizing technology breakthroughs, and incorporating the knowledge of traditional diets.

CHAPTER 4

UNRAVELING THE GLUCOSE SURGE:

Exploring the Phenomenon of Spikes

Glucose spikes are a dynamic and significant part in the complex dance that is glucose metabolism. These brief spikes in blood sugar, which are frequently disregarded, might have a significant impact on metabolic health.

Come along as we explore the complexities of glucose spikes, including their causes, effects, and preventative measures that may be taken to keep the body's glucose levels in balance.

Understanding Glucose Regulation

It is important to take a tour of the complex glucose regulation symphony, which is essential to preserving the delicate balance of blood sugar levels in the human body, before diving into the specifics of glucose spikes.

The Maestro: Insulin and Glucagon

Insulin and glucagon are two essential hormones that play a vital role in glucose management. The pancreas produces these hormones, which conduct the metabolic orchestra like maestros.

- **Insulin:** Insulin is a key player in glucose metabolism and is sometimes referred to as the director of this symphony. Insulin is released when blood sugar levels rise, usually following a carbohydrate meal. By acting as a key to open cells, it lowers blood sugar levels by enabling them to absorb glucose from the circulation.

- **Glucagon:** The antidote to insulin, glucagon is secreted when blood sugar falls. This signal instructs the liver to release glucose from stored glycogen into the circulation. By raising blood sugar levels, this procedure guarantees a steady source of energy.

Maintaining Blood Sugar Harmony

Insulin, glucagon, and other hormones must interact delicately in order for glucose control to function properly. The objective is to keep blood sugar levels within a specific range so that cells may have a constant source of energy without having too much glucose build up in the blood.

Cells and Receptors

All of the body's cells, but particularly those in the liver and muscles, are key participants in this metabolic orchestra. These cells can modify their absorption and release of glucose in response to the body's energy requirements because they include receptors that react to the signals of glucagon and insulin.

A Dynamic Harmony

The control of glucose is a dynamic feedback loop. Insulin is secreted in response to elevated blood sugar levels to promote glucose absorption and return blood sugar levels to normal. On the other hand, glucagon promotes the release of glucose that has been stored, bringing blood sugar levels back to normal.

Dietary Glucose

Dietary glucose, which comes from the carbohydrates in our food, plays a major role in the glucose symphony. The kind and time of carbohydrates affect this symphony's speed; complex carbs release glucose gradually and steadily, whereas simple sugars can cause sharp surges.

The Harmony of Hormones: Beyond Insulin and Glucagon

In addition to glucagon and insulin, a number of additional hormones are involved in the balanced control of glucose. development hormone, cortisol, and adrenaline are examples of supporting hormones that react to demands for development, physical activity, and stress.

The Conductor's Challenge: Glucose Spikes

Even with this intricate symphony, there are times when things go wrong. Glucose spikes are similar to an off-key note in a song that otherwise sounds harmonic. The conductor's capacity to keep the blood sugar levels in the delicate balance may be hampered by elements like nutrition, timing of meals, and lifestyle decisions.

The Ongoing Composition: Lifelong Metabolic Symphony

The symphony of glucose management is a continuous composition throughout life rather than a single performance. The dynamics of this symphony may alter as people age, necessitating dietary modifications, lifestyle adjustments, and maybe even pharmacological interventions to maintain the balance of blood sugar levels.

An investigation of the well choreographed dance of insulin, glucagon, cells, and hormones is necessary to comprehend glucose control. We can learn more about the processes behind the maintenance of the delicate balance of blood sugar levels—a crucial component of general health and wellbeing—by dissecting the complexities of this metabolic symphony.

The Dynamics of Glucose Spikes

Sharp increases in blood sugar levels are known as blood sugar spikes. These can happen for a number of reasons, but eating too many simple carbs is usually one of them.

This post discusses potential causes of blood sugar spikes as well as strategies for controlling blood sugar levels and averting blood sugar spikes.

What Is High Blood Sugar?

After eating, elevated blood glucose levels (hyperglycemia) happen when these levels rise above 180 mg/dL.1. A blood sugar spike is a rapid rise in blood sugar that is frequently caused by consuming an excessive amount of carbohydrate-containing meals.

Upon consuming carbohydrates containing meals, your body converts them into glucose, a simple sugar. After that, glucose gets into your blood. Your pancreas releases the hormone known as insulin in response to an increase in blood glucose levels.

The function of insulin is to operate as a key to open the doors of various bodily cells. This makes it possible for glucose to enter the cells and be stored for later use or to exit the circulation and be utilized as energy.

In the absence of insulin, glucose remains in the circulation and raises blood sugar (or glucose) levels excessively. Serious health issues may result from this.

When a person has diabetes, their insulin may occasionally be insufficient or ineffective. For this reason, it's critical that diabetics constantly check their blood sugar levels to ensure they are within a healthy range.

What Are the Symptoms of a Blood Sugar Spike?

When it occurs, some people may experience a surge in blood sugar. Usually, it happens an hour or two after eating. A blood sugar surge can cause a variety of symptoms, which might include:

- Blurry vision
- Dry mouth
- Fatigue
- Headache
- Increased thirst
- Frequent urination

Blood sugar surge symptoms can occasionally be mild and undetectable, but they are felt as the spike passes and your blood sugar falls. This may result in symptoms of low blood sugar like:

- Anxiety
- Confusion
- Dizziness
- Hunger
- Irritability

- Nervousness
- Shaking
- Sweating

Being able to identify your unique blood sugar rise symptoms can help you manage your blood sugar levels and limit any harm to your body.

Testing your blood glucose when you have these symptoms is the best technique to determine if you have diabetes or prediabetes and can spot patterns.

Speak with your healthcare practitioner about getting tested for diabetes if you do not already have the disease but exhibit symptoms of elevated blood sugar.

What Do Ketosis and Ketoacidosis Mean?

For an extended period, elevated blood sugar levels can trap glucose in the circulation, depriving your cells of energy.

Your cells start using fat as fuel when there is not enough glucose, the body's primary energy source, available. Your cells produce byproducts known as ketones when they burn fat rather than glucose for energy.

Ketone levels in diabetics who either don't produce any insulin or whose insulin isn't functioning well can rise dangerously quickly. Individuals with diabetes may have excessively acidic blood and develop diabetic ketoacidosis (DKA) if their ketone levels become too high.

Diabetic ketoacidosis is different from ketosis, the state aimed for by people following the ketogenic diet. DKA is a medical emergency and can result in diabetic coma or death.

Symptoms of Diabetic Ketoacidosis

Call 911 or seek medical attention immediately if you experience any signs or symptoms of DKA, such as:

- Confusion and decreased alertness
- Dehydration, dry skin, and severely dry mouth
- Flushed face
- Frequent urination
- Fruity smelling breath
- Headache
- Loss of consciousness
- Muscle stiffness
- Nausea and vomiting

- Rapid breathing
- Stomach pain
- Weakness

What Are the Causes of Blood Sugar Spikes?

Your blood sugar levels will normally rise and fall throughout the day as your body alternates between fed and unfed states. Insulin and stored glycogen control blood sugar levels in healthy individuals to keep them within normal ranges.

Those with diabetes are more likely than those without the disease to have a surge in blood sugar. Blood sugar spikes are mostly caused by eating meals high in simple carbs, such as bread and pasta made from refined grains, sweetened drinks, and sweets.

However, there are additional causes for high blood sugar levels, such as:

- Eating more than planned
- Exercising less than planned
- Not taking enough diabetes medication (oral or injectable) or needing changes to your medication dosage
- Illness or infection
- Having an injury or recent surgery
- Stress
- Taking certain medications, such as steroids
- Over-treating low blood sugar levels
- Dehydration

Early morning blood sugar spikes, which result in high fasting blood sugar, can be caused by:

Dawn phenomenon: This is an early-morning blood sugar spike that occurs naturally. Insulin-resistant diabetes may have greater levels of it.

Somogyi effect: This is a result of low blood sugar levels in the middle of the night and your body producing hormones to boost blood sugar levels, which is why your blood sugar levels are high in the early morning.

How to Manage Blood Sugar

Blood sugar self-management is a crucial part of diabetes treatment. If you have diabetes, it's imperative that you understand how to address elevated and lowered blood sugar levels. Here are some pointers for controlling your blood sugar levels correctly.

1. Proper Hydration

It's still crucial to stay hydrated even if you don't have diabetes. The majority of the body is made of water, which is also essential to several bodily processes. Water is essential to life for a variety of reasons, including food absorption and digestion, joint lubrication, and body temperature regulation.

Dehydration can lead to a concentration of blood sugar in diabetics, which can spike blood sugar levels.

You can meet the majority of your daily fluid requirements by drinking water throughout the day. Fruits and vegetables, among other foods, contain water that contributes to your daily water consumption. Drink water instead of sugar-sweetened liquids including juice, sports drinks, soft drinks, sweet tea, and flavored coffee beverages.

Follow these tips for drinking more water:

- Keep a water bottle nearby and refill it throughout the day.
- Make infused water by adding slices of fresh fruit, vegetables, or herbs to your water.
- Drink sparkling water with a splash of 100% fruit juice.
- Ask for water when dining out.
- Keep a pitcher of water in the refrigerator to always have cold water to drink.

2. Meal Timing

When it comes to controlling blood sugar levels, timing of meals might be just as crucial as content. Blood sugar fluctuations can be avoided by eating at regular times. Maintain a consistent eating routine by having the same number of meals and snacks at the same time every day.

This may take the form of five to six smaller meals spread out throughout the day, or it could look like three conventional meals with two to three snacks in between. Select the method that suits you the most and stay with it.

High Blood Sugar at Night and What to Do About It

1. Relaxation Techniques

Learning how to relax and de-stress will assist lower blood sugar levels since stress hormones can elevate blood sugar levels. Something that one person finds soothing could make another feel more anxious. Investigate several approaches and strategies to assist with stress management. Discover what suits you best.

Some examples include:

- Meditation
- Deep breathing
- Progressive muscle relaxation (alternating tension and relaxation in the major muscle groups)

- Journal writing
- Going for a walk
- Reading a book
- Yoga
- Listening to calming music
- Taking a warm bath

2 . Better Sleep

Getting a good night's sleep every night can lower the risk of obesity and stress hormones. To help you maintain a regular sleep and wake time and to help regulate your circadian rhythm, try to get seven to nine hours of sleep every night.

Consider these additional tips for getting better sleep:

- Put away electronics, such as cell phones and TV, at least an hour before bedtime.

- Limit daytime naps.
- Keep a calm and restful sleeping environment.
- Participate in physical activity throughout the day.
- Avoid caffeine late in the day.

3 . Physical Activity

Engaging in physical exercise can improve insulin sensitivity, which will improve its ability to lower blood sugar levels. Aim for 150 minutes a week of moderate exercise.

Start modestly if it has been a long since you last exercised. Make an effort to get in 15 to 20 minutes of activity every day, or split it up into three 10-minute sessions. Choose activities that you love and can maintain, and move your body in ways that make you happy.

Medication

You can control your diabetes and prevent blood sugar spikes by taking medication. Diabetes treatments come in two primary forms: injectables and oral (pills).

Your prescription regimen will be determined by a number of variables, including the kind of diabetes you have, your medical history, how well your diabetes is being managed right now, and any additional drugs you may be taking. Aim to take your medicine as prescribed by your doctor, and never stop taking it without first talking to them.

How to Prevent Blood Sugar Spikes

There are additional ways to prevent blood sugar spikes.

Monitor blood sugar levels: Finding out what your initial blood sugar levels are is the first step towards avoiding blood sugar spikes. You should check your blood sugar level frequently, especially if you take medicine like insulin that directly affects it.

Check your blood sugar level every morning before you eat: This blood sugar level is known as a fasting level. For certain type 2 diabetics, this once-daily testing may be enough. Others, meanwhile, could require up to 10 daily blood sugar checks.

Choose whole grains: Whole grains, as opposed to refined grains, are composed of the complete grain, including the nutrient-rich inner core known as the germ and the fibrous outer coating known as the bran. You will obtain the most amount of nutrients from your grains if you choose to consume whole grains.

Eat more fiber: Fiber doesn't cause a significant rise in blood sugar since it isn't absorbed and processed by the body in the same way as other carbs.

Balance meals with fat and protein: Eating fat and protein together with carbs can help reduce the risk of blood sugar rises. Carbohydrates rapidly convert to glucose when consumed by themselves, causing a blood sugar increase. Carbohydrate absorption into the circulation is slowed down with the assistance of fat and protein.

Long-term side effects

Long-term increased blood sugar levels are usually the cause of problems related to diabetes mellitus. Before symptoms manifest, diabetes problems may develop gradually over a number of years.

The risk of major consequences from diabetes, such as heart disease, blindness, neuropathy, and renal failure, is increased in people with chronically high blood sugar.

Untreated hyperglycemia may potentially progress to ketoacidosis. This is a serious condition that may result in mortality or a diabetic coma.

Long-term elevated blood sugar levels might have an impact on your major organs and bodily systems.

Other complications of diabetes can include:

Eye problems

Diabetes increases a person's chance of acquiring eye issues, such as:

- cataracts
- retinopathy
- glaucoma

A cataract is an opacification and thickening of the eye's lens that can cause blurriness and reduce night vision.

Diabetic retinopathy is a condition where abnormal growth of tiny blood vessels causes damage to the retina's blood vessels. This abnormal growth is thought to be associated with long-term untreated high blood sugar levels. Although symptoms may not show up right away, they can eventually cause blindness.

An elevated risk of glaucoma can result from diabetic retinopathy. This illness results in an accumulation of pressure within the eye, which reduces blood flow and damages the optic nerve and retina.

Kidney disease

The progressive kidney condition known as diabetic nephropathy causes the kidneys, which are in charge of filtering the body's waste, to fail. It occurs when the kidneys' blood arteries are harmed by elevated blood sugar levels.

Renal failure can develop from kidney disease, even though you may not have symptoms at the beginning.

Nerve damage (diabetic neuropathy)

One of the most dangerous consequences of diabetes is diabetic neuropathy, or nerve damage. Long-term elevated blood sugar levels are the root cause of it.

Most symptoms start off slowly and progress over several decades.

There are four main types of neuropathy that affect people with diabetes:

- peripheral neuropathy

- autonomic neuropathy
- proximal neuropathy
- focal neuropathy

Heart and blood vessel diseases

High blood sugar levels have the potential to harm your heart's blood vessels and nerves over time. Diabetes also raises a person's risk of cardiovascular illnesses, such as heart attacks and strokes.

Blood vessel blockage can also occur from untreated high blood sugar. Foot ulcers and infections may result from this. It may result in the amputation of a lower limb, foot, or toe in extreme circumstances.

Periodontal disease

Diabetes increases a person's chance of acquiring periodontal disease, often known as gum disease.
Elevated blood sugar levels can cause the mouth to produce more sugar, which can harm dental health in general. Diabetes increases the risk of increased plaque production, decreased salivary flow, and impaired gum circulation.

Reaching and keeping glucose balance is like playing a well-balanced symphony. It entails a complex interaction between lifestyle decisions, nutritional choices, and an awareness of personal reactions. Understanding the nuances of glucose spikes and using balancing techniques can help people move toward metabolic equilibrium and long-term health and wellbeing.

Investigating glucose spikes reveals a dynamic facet of metabolic health, highlighting the significance of lifestyle behaviors and well-informed decision-making in preserving balance. As we work through the complexity of this phenomena, we learn things that enable us to work with our bodies to create a symphony of health.

CHAPTER 5

THE TRIAD OF EFFECTS

Deconstructing the Three Consequences of Glucose Spikes

The implications of glucose spikes are a trio of effects that echo throughout the body within the complex symphony of glucose metabolism.

These effects, which range from short-term physiological reactions to long-term ramifications, demonstrate the complex effects of brief increases in blood sugar. To comprehend the complex interactions between these impacts, let us dissect the trio.

Insulin Resistance: A Crescendo of Metabolic Disruption

The pancreas produces insulin during glucose rises to help cells absorb glucose. On the other hand, a crescendo of the insulin response occurs with prolonged or numerous increases.

As a result of the constant need for insulin, cells may become more sensitive. Insulin resistance is the term for the process by which cells lose their ability to respond to the effects of insulin over time.

The delicate ballet of glucose management is thrown off balance by insulin resistance. Insulin signals are resisted by cells, which prevents glucose from being absorbed efficiently and creates the conditions for persistently high blood sugar.

Inflammation: The Harmonic Discord in Metabolic Harmony

Spikes in blood sugar, particularly when coupled with insulin resistance, can exacerbate an inflammatory milieu in the body.

Inflammatory pathways are activated by elevated blood sugar. This persistent low-grade inflammation aggravates the problems caused by insulin resistance and tampers with regular regulatory functions.

Within the metabolic symphony, inflammation becomes a harmonizing dissonance that accelerates the development of metabolic diseases and raises the risk of cardiovascular problems and other health consequences.

Energy Fluctuations: The Staccato Rhythm of Peaks and Valleys

The body's energy availability is characterized by staccato rhythms caused by spikes in glucose levels followed by subsequent dips.

Following a surge, a sharp decline in blood sugar levels may cause feelings of exhaustion, agitation, and a need for faster energy sources.

The erratic energy levels cause a cycle of highs and lows, interfering with the constant energy supply required for the best possible physical and mental performance.

The Interplay of Consequences: A Symphony of Metabolic Challenges

Insulin resistance, inflammation, and energy swings interact to produce a metabolic symphony that intensifies each other.

Both inflammation and insulin resistance are factors in energy imbalances. The interaction of these effects paves the way for the emergence and advancement of metabolic diseases, including type 2 diabetes and heart problems.

The trio of consequences materializes as a continuous performance, with one effect amplifying and impacting the others. An all-encompassing strategy to address the underlying causes of glucose spikes and their knock-on consequences is needed to break this cycle.

The trio of consequences arising from elevated glucose levels constitutes a symphony of metabolic obstacles. Long-term health is impacted by a complex interplay between insulin resistance, inflammation, and energy swings that goes beyond acute physiological reactions. Comprehending and resolving these outcomes are essential measures for arranging a balanced metabolic balance and promoting general health.

CHAPTER 6

MASTERING THE ART OF BLOOD SUGAR BALANCE

Strategies to Level Your Glucose Curve

Achieving a stable and balanced glucose curve is like learning the skill of a harmonic performance in the complex dance of glucose metabolism. Blood sugar regulation is a dynamic process that calls for deliberate lifestyle decisions and strategy implementation.

Together, we can determine practical measures to help you achieve optimal metabolic health and level your glucose curve.

Harmony in Nutrition: Crafting a Balanced Plate

Embrace Whole Foods: Select full, nutrient-dense foods such as lean meats, healthy fats, whole grains, and a range of fruits and vegetables. These meals release glucose gradually, avoiding sudden surges.

Opt for Complex Carbohydrates: Give complex carbs—like those found in whole grains, legumes, and veggies—priority over refined and processed carbohydrates. The slower glucose release from these carbs encourages sustained energy levels.

Balance Macronutrients: Make sure that every meal has an equal amount of fats, proteins, and carbs. This mixture promotes general metabolic health and regulates the absorption of glucose.

Timed Symphonies: The Rhythm of Meal Timing

Regular Meal Times: To develop a rhythmic pattern for glucose management, set regular meal times. Meal time that is consistent aids the body in better anticipating and controlling glucose levels.

Smart Snacking: Eat well-balanced snacks in between meals to keep your energy levels constant. To prevent unexpected glucose spikes, choose foods that blend carbs with proteins or good fats.

Mindful Eating Practices: Eat mindfully by observing your body's hunger signals, taking your time, and not rushing through meals. This strategy helps avoid overeating and promotes improved digestion.

Exercise: The Dynamic Movement in Glucose Regulation

Regular Physical Activity: Exercise on a regular basis, combining strength training and aerobic activity. Exercise improves insulin sensitivity, which improves the way cells use glucose.

Post-Meal Walks: After eating, especially a substantial one, take brisk walking. By promoting glucose absorption into cells, this easy exercise lowers postprandial glucose levels.

Find Enjoyable Activities: To ensure that exercising remains a sustainable part of your routine, choose activities you love. This enhances glucose metabolism and improves general health at the same time.

Hydration: The Fluidity of Metabolic Support

Stay Hydrated: Sufficient hydration promotes proper glucose control as well as general metabolic activity. Water is necessary for several physiological functions, one of which is the breakdown of carbohydrates.

Limit Sugary Drinks: Sugar-filled drinks should be avoided since they might cause sharp rises in blood sugar. Choose water, herbal teas, or other sugar-free, low-calorie drinks.

Balanced Electrolytes: Maintain an equilibrium of electrolytes since they are essential for healthy metabolic processes and cellular hydration.

Stress Management: The Melody of Emotional Well-Being

Mind-Body Practices: Include stress-relieving techniques like yoga, deep breathing, and meditation. Prolonged stress can lead to high cortisol levels, which can affect how the body uses glucose.

Adequate Sleep: Give adequate, high-quality sleep first priority. Lack of sleep can throw off the hormonal balance, which can impact glucose control and insulin sensitivity.

Work-Life Balance: Aim for a balanced work-life schedule to reduce long-term pressures. Define limits and schedule enjoyable and restorative activities.

Monitoring and Adjusting: The Conductor's Vigilance

Regular Glucose Monitoring: If necessary, keep a close eye on your blood sugar levels, particularly if you suffer from diabetes or another related ailment. You may use this knowledge to make well-informed decisions and modify your lifestyle as necessary.

Consultation with Healthcare Professionals: Consult medical experts, such as endocrinologists and qualified dietitians, for advice. They are able to offer tailored advice according to your particular medical requirements.

Adaptation to Changes: Be flexible and prepared to modify your tactics as necessary. Your body's reaction to certain lifestyle modifications might be influenced by factors including age, exercise level, and health issues.

Gaining proficiency in glucose control balancing requires a comprehensive strategy that incorporates timing, exercise, diet, hydration, stress reduction, and close observation. You may empower yourself to level your glucose curve, support a healthy metabolic symphony, and promote long-term wellbeing by putting these techniques into practice.

CHAPTER 7

DIABETES NUTRITIONAL GUIDE

What is the glycemic index (GI)?

One nutritional measure you may use to assess the quality of the carbohydrates you eat is the glycemic index (GI).

The speed at which the carbohydrates in a particular diet affect your blood sugar is measured by the glycemic index.

Based on how rapidly a food raises your blood sugar level in comparison to glucose or white bread (which have a glycemic index value of 100), items are labeled low, medium, or high on the glycemic index.

Selecting foods with a low glycemic index will help you reduce sharp spikes in your blood sugar.

Consuming a food with a high glycemic index will also likely cause your blood sugar to rise more sharply. A higher blood sugar measurement after a meal may also result from it.

A food's glycemic index can vary depending on a number of factors. These elements consist of the food's ingredients and cooking method. Combining different foods also affects a food's glycemic index.

A typical portion of a certain dish is not the basis for calculating a food's glycemic index. Carrots, for instance, have a high glycemic index, but you would need to consume a pound and a half to reach the threshold.

There is also another measurement that is available, known as glycemic load.

This measurement accounts for the rate of food digestion as well as the quantity found in a typical dish. This might be a more accurate method of determining how a food high in carbohydrates affects blood sugar.

What factors affect a food's glycemic index rating?

Foods are categorized into three groups in order to receive a GI number: low, medium, or high.

- Low GI foods have a GI of 55 or less.
- Medium GI foods are between 56 and 69.
- High GI foods are 70 or higher.

Glycemic load is categorized as low (less than 10), medium (between 10 and 20), and high (more than 20).

The process of determining a food's glycemic rating takes several elements into consideration.

These factors include:

Acidity

Pickles and other highly acidic foods have a tendency to be lower on the GI scale than lower on it. This explains why lactic acid-based foods, like sourdough bread, have a lower GI than white bread.

Cooking Time

Food often has a higher GI the longer it is cooked. Starch or carbs begin to break down when food is cooked.

Fiber Content

Foods high in fiber typically have lower glycemic ratings.

Because beans and seeds have fibrous coats around them, the body breaks them down more slowly. As such, their glycemic index is often lower than that of meals without this coating.

Processing

In general, a food's glycemic index increases with its level of processing. Fruit juice, for instance, is GI-rated higher than raw fruit.

Ripeness

A fruit or vegetable's tendency to be higher on the GI is correlated with how ripe it is.

These are some broad parameters to consider when assessing a food's possible influence on blood sugar, however there are undoubtedly exceptions to every rule.

How does one apply the Glycemic Index?

You may more effectively control your post-meal blood sugar levels by eating in accordance with the GI. You can also get assistance from the GI in choosing the right dietary combinations.

Eating multiple low GI fruits and vegetables in conjunction with a high GI item, for example, will help you maintain better blood sugar management. Other ideas include combining beans with rice, nut butter with toast, and tomato sauce with spaghetti.

What are the benefits of using the glycemic index?

Low-glycemic meals are a good way to maintain low blood sugar levels. But you also have to pay close attention to the suggested portion proportions. Glycemic scores are not limited to those with diabetes.

The GI diet is also used by those who are seeking to reduce their appetite or lose weight since it can regulate hunger. A person may feel fuller for longer since the meal takes longer for the body to digest.

What are the risks of eating on the glycemic index?

Glycemic index: It assists you in selecting better-quality carbs. Nevertheless, the ultimate factor influencing blood sugar levels is the overall amount of carbohydrates in your diet.

Selecting meals with low glycemic index can be beneficial, but controlling the amount of carbs you eat is also necessary.

Furthermore, the GI does not account for a food's whole nutritional content. For example, you shouldn't subsist only on microwave popcorn simply because it's included in the group of GI foods.

The American Diabetes Association advises consulting a licensed dietitian with experience in managing diabetes when beginning a diet.

There are several options for food programs. Make sure to inquire about the ideal ways to utilize the glycemic index facts to regulate your blood sugar level.

The glycemic index of common fruits and vegetables

Maintaining a nutritious diet is essential for managing diabetes. Vegetables and fruits are essential components of a balanced diet.

You may pick your favorites to include in your daily diet by being aware of the glycemic load and glycemic index of some of the more popular fruits and vegetables.

The Harvard Health Publication lists them as follows:

Fruits	Glycemic index (glucose = 100)	Serving size (grams)	Glycemic load per serving
Apple, average	39	120	6
Banana, ripe	62	120	16

Dates, dried	42	80	18
Grapefruit	25	120	3
Grapes, average	59	120	11

Orange, average	40	120	4
Peach, average	42	120	5
Peach, canned in light syrup	40	120	5

Pear, average	43	120	5
Pear, canned in pear juice	38	120	4
Prunes, pitted	29	60	10

Raisins	64	60	28
Watermelon	72	120	4

Vegetables	Glycemic index (glucose = 100)	Serving size (grams)	Glycemic load per serving
Green peas, average	51	80	4
Carrots, average	35	80	2

Parsnips	52	80	4
Baked russet potato, average	111	150	33
Boiled white potato, average	82	150	21

Instant mashed potato, average	87	150	17
Sweet potato, average	70	150	22
Yam, average	54	150	20

Takeaway

You will be able to better control your blood sugar levels if you utilize the glycemic index to plan your meals. Additionally, you'll be able to locate and select meals that you like. After that, you may include them in a nutritious diet.

Dietary management of blood sugar levels is a critical component of diabetes management.

I WISH YOU A HEALTHY LIFE.

Printed in Great Britain
by Amazon